TABLE OF CONTENTS

CHAPTER 1: THE INTERPLAY OF WORK AND FITNESS

- Understanding the interconnectedness between work and physical well-being.

- Exploring how each aspect influences the other in our daily lives.

- Setting the stage for a holistic approach to balance.

In our modern lives, the demands of work and the pursuit of physical well-being are often seen as competing priorities. However, they are deeply interconnected, each influencing the other in profound ways. Understanding this relationship is key to achieving a balanced and sustainable lifestyle.

1. Understanding the Interconnectedness

The tapestry of our lives intricately weaves together our work and fitness, each thread influencing the strength and pattern of the other. Our job demands, work environment, and daily routines are the loom on which our lifestyle is crafted. When work pressures mount, they can tug at the threads of our physical fitness, leading to a fraying of our overall well-being.

The consequences of neglecting fitness due to work are manifold —diminished health, decreased energy levels, and a potential increase in stress-related ailments.

Work and physical fitness are not isolated aspects of our lives; they constantly interact and impact each other. Consider how the demands of your job affect your ability to prioritize exercise and healthy habits.

Long hours, stressful deadlines, and sedentary desk work can all hinder our efforts to stay active and healthy. Acknowledging this interconnectedness is the first step toward creating harmony between work and fitness.

2. Exploring Mutual Influences

The influence of work on physical fitness and vice versa is significant. For instance, prolonged sitting at a desk can lead to poor posture, muscle tension, and weight gain. Conversely, regular exercise can enhance focus, reduce stress, and boost overall productivity at work.

Delve into real-life examples and studies that highlight these mutual influences to underscore the importance of striking a balance.

The relationship between work and fitness is bidirectional. Sedentary desk jobs, for example, can lead to a lifestyle marked by physical inactivity, which is a known risk factor for various health issues.

High-stress work environments can take a toll on mental health, reducing one's energy levels and motivation to engage in physical activity. On the flip side, maintaining a regular fitness routine can have a positive impact on work performance.

Exercise is known to improve cognitive function, productivity, and stress management—benefits that are reflected in one's professional life.

3. Setting the Stage for Holistic Balance

To achieve true harmony between work and physical fitness, we must adopt a holistic approach. This entails addressing not only the physical aspects of health but also the mental and emotional components. Share practical strategies for integrating fitness into daily work routines, such as incorporating short movement breaks, practicing mindfulness techniques, or optimizing workspace ergonomics.

Achieving harmony between work and fitness requires a holistic approach that encompasses the physical, mental, and emotional aspects of our well-being. Here are some practical strategies to integrate fitness into daily work routines:

Incorporate Short Movement Breaks

Set a timer to remind yourself to stand up and move every hour. Even a few minutes of stretching, walking, or simple exercises can counteract the effects of prolonged sitting.

Practice Mindfulness Techniques

Dedicate moments in your day for mindfulness practices such as deep breathing, meditation, or guided imagery. These techniques can reduce stress and increase focus, enhancing both mental and physical health.

Optimize Workspace Ergonomics

Arrange your workspace to promote good posture and reduce strain. Consider an adjustable chair, an ergonomic keyboard, or a standing desk to support your physical health while you work.

Engage in Regular Exercise

Schedule regular exercise sessions into your calendar as you would any important meeting. Whether it's a morning jog, a lunchtime yoga class, or an evening workout, make it a non-negotiable part of your routine.

Healthy Eating Habits

Prepare nutritious meals and snacks that fuel your body and mind. Opt for whole foods rich in nutrients and avoid excessive caffeine and sugar that can lead to energy crashes.

Quality Sleep

Prioritize getting enough quality sleep each night. Good sleep is essential for recovery, performance, and overall health.

Social Support

Build a support network of colleagues, friends, or online communities who share your commitment to balancing work and fitness. They can offer encouragement, share tips, and help you stay accountable.

CHAPTER 2: REDEFINING PRODUCTIVITY

- Challenging traditional notions of productivity and success.

- Introducing the concept of holistic productivity that encompasses both work and fitness goals.

- Strategies for aligning productivity with well-being.

In a world driven by deadlines and output, it's time to rethink our approach to productivity. True productivity goes beyond mere task completion; it encompasses overall well-being and the pursuit of balanced success.

In today's fast-paced world, the traditional metrics of productivity—deadlines met, tasks completed, hours logged—no longer suffice. True productivity is not just about the output; it's about the outcome and the quality of life it brings. It's about redefining success to include well-being, balance, and personal fulfillment.

1. Challenging Traditional Notions of Productivity and Success

The traditional workplace often glorifies the grind—long hours and constant output—as the path to success. However, this narrow view of productivity can lead to serious drawbacks:

Burnout: The relentless push for output can result in chronic stress and burnout, leaving individuals exhausted and unable to perform at their best.

Neglect of Personal Health: When work takes precedence, personal health often takes a backseat. This neglect can manifest as poor nutrition, lack of exercise, and inadequate sleep, all of which can have long-term negative effects on one's health.

Diminished Creativity: A workaholic mindset leaves little room for the rest and relaxation that the brain needs to foster creativity. Without downtime, our ability to innovate and problem-solve is significantly impaired.

Beyond Task Completion

The relentless pursuit of task completion can lead to a myopic view of what it means to be productive. Instead, we should consider:

Quality Over Quantity: The value of our work should not be measured solely by how much we do but by the impact and quality of what we accomplish.

Sustainable Practices: Long-term productivity is about creating sustainable habits that support our health, creativity, and ability to innovate.

Well-being as a Priority: A truly productive individual is not just efficient at work but also enjoys a state of well-being that encompasses physical health, mental clarity, and emotional stability.

The Pursuit of Balanced Success

Balanced success means aligning our professional achievements with our personal values and well-being. It involves:

Setting Boundaries: Knowing when to step back and recharge is crucial for maintaining productivity without burnout.

Holistic Goal-Setting: Goals should reflect not only career aspirations but also personal development and health.

Mindfulness and Reflection: Regularly reflecting on our work and its alignment with our life goals ensures that we stay on a path that is meaningful and fulfilling.

Redefining productivity is a call to action—to shift our focus from mere efficiency to a more holistic view of success. It's about building a life where our work supports our well-being, and our well-being enhances our work.

Challenging Traditional Notions of Productivity and Success

In the quest for professional achievement, society often heralds the relentless pursuit of more: more hours, more tasks, more output. This conventional definition of productivity equates to a state of constant work, often glorified as workaholism. However, this narrow perspective overlooks the significant drawbacks of such a mindset:

Burnout: The incessant drive for productivity can lead to an overwhelming sense of exhaustion and a loss of enthusiasm for work, known as burnout. This state not only diminishes an individual's capacity to perform but also affects their overall quality of life.

In the relentless pursuit of efficiency, we've been conditioned to measure success by the volume of tasks we complete. Yet, this narrow focus on constant output and workaholism has significant drawbacks. It leads to burnout, neglect of personal health, and diminished creativity.

We must encourage a paradigm shift, urging readers to reassess their own definitions of success and productivity. It's essential to include holistic well-being in this new definition, recognizing that a truly productive life is not just about what we do but also about how we feel while doing it.

It's time to encourage a shift in perspective. We must question the conventional definitions of productivity and success that prioritize constant output over well-being. Readers are urged to reassess their own definitions of success and productivity to include holistic well-being. This includes:

Mental Health: Recognizing the importance of mental health in the productivity equation.

Physical Health: Understanding that a healthy body supports a productive mind.

Emotional Well-being: Acknowledging that emotional resilience is foundational to sustained success.

By broadening our definition of productivity to encompass these aspects of well-being, we pave the way for a more sustainable and fulfilling path to success.

2. Introducing Holistic Productivity

Holistic productivity is a transformative approach that integrates work and fitness goals, creating a synergy between professional achievements and personal well-being. It's a comprehensive strategy that recognizes the interdependence of various aspects of our lives.

The Pillars of Holistic Productivity:

Physical Health: Regular exercise, adequate sleep, and proper nutrition are not just good for the body; they enhance cognitive function and workplace performance.

Mental Health: Mindfulness practices, stress management, and work-life boundaries contribute to a resilient and focused mind.

Emotional Well-being: Emotional intelligence and healthy social interactions are crucial for a supportive and productive work environment.

Enhancing Productivity Through Healthy Habits:

Routine Exercise: Incorporating physical activity into your daily routine boosts energy levels and increases mental clarity.

Balanced Diet: A diet rich in nutrients supports brain health and has been linked to improved concentration and decision-making abilities.

Quality Sleep: Prioritizing sleep is essential for recovery and performance. A well-rested mind is more efficient and innovative.

Neglect of Personal Health: A work-centric lifestyle often comes at the expense of personal health. Neglecting nutrition, sleep, and exercise in favor of work can have detrimental effects on both physical and mental well-being.

Diminished Creativity: Creativity thrives in environments that allow for rest, reflection, and diverse experiences. A fixation on constant output can stifle creative thought, limiting one's ability to innovate and solve problems effectively.

It's time to encourage a reevaluation of what it means to be productive and successful. True productivity should encompass a holistic view of well-being, where success is not just measured by work output but also by the quality of one's health, happiness, and life satisfaction.

Encouraging Holistic Well-being:

Mental and Emotional Health: Recognize the importance of mental and emotional well-being as integral components of productivity. Practices such as mindfulness and regular breaks can support a healthier work-life balance.

Physical Health: Emphasize the role of physical health in maintaining productivity. Regular exercise, proper nutrition, and adequate sleep are foundational to sustaining energy and focus.

Creative and Social Fulfillment: Acknowledge the value of creative pursuits and social connections. Engaging in hobbies and spending time with loved ones can rejuvenate the spirit and inspire new ideas.

By broadening our definition of productivity to include these aspects of well-being, we pave the way for a more sustainable and fulfilling path to success.

Setting Balanced Goals:

SMART Goals: Goals should be Specific, Measurable, Achievable, Relevant, and Time-bound, with a balance between work objectives and personal health.

Integrated Goal Planning: When setting professional targets, consider how they align with personal well-being. For example, a goal to enhance leadership skills could be paired with a commitment to mindfulness training.

Regular Review and Adjustment: Life is dynamic, and so should be our goals. Regularly reviewing and adjusting goals ensures they remain aligned with personal values and well-being.

Holistic productivity is not about doing more; it's about doing better. By adopting healthy habits and setting balanced goals, we can enhance our productivity in a sustainable and fulfilling way.

3. Strategies for Aligning Productivity with Well-being

To align productivity with well-being, consider the following practical strategies:

Time Blocking: Allocate dedicated time slots for work, exercise, and rest to maintain a balanced schedule. This ensures that each aspect of your life receives the attention it deserves.

Prioritization: Identify key tasks that contribute to long-term goals. Delegate or eliminate non-essential activities to focus on what truly matters.

Mindful Work Practices: Incorporate mindfulness techniques into work routines to enhance focus and reduce stress. This could be as simple as taking deep breaths before starting a new task.

Physical Activity Breaks: Encourage regular movement breaks during work hours to boost energy and creativity. Even a short walk can reinvigorate the mind.

Goal Setting: Set SMART (Specific, Measurable, Achievable, Relevant, Time-bound) goals that encompass both work and fitness objectives. This holistic approach ensures that your goals are balanced and attainable.

3. Strategies for Aligning Productivity with Well-being

To align productivity with well-being, consider the following practical strategies:

Time Blocking: Allocate dedicated time slots for work, exercise, and rest to maintain a balanced schedule. This ensures that each aspect of your life receives the attention it deserves.

Time blocking is a method of scheduling your day into segments where you focus on specific tasks or groups of tasks. This technique helps prevent multitasking and ensures that both work and personal time are respected. For example, you might block off mornings for deep work, afternoons for meetings, and evenings for family and relaxation.

Prioritization: Identify key tasks that contribute to long-term goals. Delegate or eliminate non-essential activities to focus on what truly matters.

Prioritization involves identifying the most important tasks that will have the greatest impact on your goals. Use tools like the Eisenhower Matrix to categorize tasks by urgency and importance, focusing on what truly moves you forward.

Mindful Work Practices: Incorporate mindfulness techniques into work routines to enhance focus and reduce stress. This could be as simple as taking deep breaths before starting a new task.

Incorporate mindful work practices such as meditation, deep breathing, or taking short pauses to refocus throughout the day. These practices can enhance concentration, reduce stress, and improve overall job satisfaction.

Physical Activity Breaks: Encourage regular movement breaks during work hours to boost energy and creativity. Even a short walk can reinvigorate the mind.

Regular physical activity breaks during the workday can increase energy levels and creativity. This could be as simple as a five-minute stretch, a walk around the block, or a quick workout session.

Goal Setting: Set SMART (Specific, Measurable, Achievable, Relevant, Time-bound) goals that encompass both work and fitness objectives. This holistic approach ensures that your goals are balanced and attainable.

Set SMART goals (Specific, Measurable, Achievable, Relevant, Time-bound) that encompass both professional and personal objectives. This holistic approach ensures that your goals are balanced and contribute to your overall well-being.

CHAPTER 3: EMBRACING FLEXIBILITY

- The importance of flexibility in both work and fitness routines.

- Techniques for adapting to changing circumstances and schedules.

- Finding balance through fluidity and adaptability.

1. The Importance of Flexibility in Work and Fitness Routines

In our fast-paced world, the ability to adapt is invaluable. Flexibility in work and fitness routines allows individuals to navigate the unpredictable demands of life with grace and resilience. Rigid schedules and inflexible expectations can be a recipe for stress and frustration, leading to a decrease in productivity and a negative impact on health.

Flexibility, on the other hand, fosters a culture of innovation and personal growth.

It allows for adjustments in response to unforeseen circumstances and enables individuals to maintain their fitness goals even amidst a hectic work schedule. This adaptability is not about compromising on objectives; it's about finding creative ways to achieve them without sacrificing well-being.

Adaptable routines encourage a proactive rather than reactive approach to challenges, leading to improved overall productivity and health. By embracing flexibility, we open ourselves to new opportunities and ways of thinking that can significantly enhance our quality of life.

This section emphasizes the importance of flexibility in both professional and personal realms, advocating for a more adaptable and fluid approach to daily routines for enhanced productivity and well-being.

Flexibility—the quality of bending easily without breaking—is often associated with physical fitness. However, its significance extends far beyond the physical realm into how we manage our work and personal lives. Flexibility in our routines and mindsets is becoming increasingly essential in a world that is constantly changing and presenting new challenges.

Navigating the Demands of Work

In the workplace, flexibility can mean the difference between thriving and merely surviving. Rigid schedules and inflexible expectations can lead to a buildup of stress and frustration, as they leave little room for the unexpected or for personal needs. On the other hand, flexibility allows for adjustments that can lead to greater satisfaction and effectiveness. It enables innovation, as employees who feel free to adapt their approach can come up with creative solutions to problems.

Maintaining Fitness Goals

Similarly, when it comes to maintaining fitness goals, a flexible approach is key. Life can be unpredictable, and rigid workout schedules can quickly become untenable. Flexibility allows us to adjust our fitness routines to fit our changing circumstances, ensuring that we stay on track even when life gets busy or complicated.

Benefits of Adaptable Routines

Adaptable routines have numerous benefits for overall productivity and health:

Reduced Stress: Flexibility in scheduling helps mitigate stress by accommodating life's uncertainties.

Increased Productivity: By allowing for adjustments, flexible routines can lead to more efficient use of time and resources.

Improved Health: Flexibility in managing work and fitness can lead to better health outcomes by reducing the risk of burnout and providing opportunities to incorporate healthy activities into our daily lives.

Flexibility is not about sacrificing goals or lowering standards; it's about finding smarter, more sustainable ways to achieve them. By embracing flexibility, we can create a more balanced and fulfilling approach to work and life.

2. Techniques for Adapting to Changing Circumstances

Adaptability is the cornerstone of a flexible approach to life. Here are some practical techniques to weave flexibility into the fabric of our daily routines:

Time Management: Effective time management is pivotal in adapting to unexpected changes. Prioritization and time blocking are not about restricting freedom but about creating a structure that can flexibly accommodate new priorities as they arise. By categorizing tasks based on urgency and importance, we can ensure that our energy is directed toward the most impactful activities.

Prioritization and time blocking are key to managing unexpected changes. By determining what needs to be done and when, you can create a flexible schedule that allows for the unexpected. This might involve setting aside specific times for focused work and other times for potential interruptions or new opportunities.

Alternative Workspaces: The traditional office is no longer the sole workspace option. Remote work and co-working spaces offer the flexibility to choose environments that best support our diverse work styles. These alternatives can lead to increased productivity and satisfaction by allowing us to work in settings that resonate with our personal preferences and professional needs.

Fitness Adaptations: Our fitness routines need not be rigid. When faced with time constraints, travel, or physical limitations, we can adapt our workouts to fit our circumstances. This might mean shorter, more intense workouts, using bodyweight exercises when away from the gym, or finding creative ways to incorporate physical activity into our day.

Mindset Shifts: Cultivating a mindset of resilience and openness to change is perhaps the most important aspect of flexibility. This mindset allows you to see change as an opportunity rather than a setback, fostering creativity and problem-solving abilities. It involves being proactive in learning new skills and adapting to new situations.

By adopting these techniques, you can build a life that is resilient to change and open to the opportunities that come with it.

3. Finding Balance Through Fluidity and Adaptability

Embracing flexibility is key to finding balance in our hectic lives and enhancing overall well-being.

Embracing flexibility is akin to moving with the rhythm of life, allowing for a dance between structure and spontaneity that leads to greater balance and well-being.

Reduced Stress: Flexibility acts as a buffer against the rigidity of strict routines and deadlines. By promoting a more relaxed approach to work and fitness, it allows for a breathing space where individuals can recalibrate and refocus. This reduction in pressure can lead to lower stress levels, making room for a more enjoyable and sustainable way of living.

Flexibility can significantly reduce the pressure that comes from strict routines and deadlines. By allowing for a more relaxed approach to work and fitness, we can adapt to life's demands without the added stress of rigid schedules. This adaptability can lead to a calmer, more centered existence, where unexpected events are managed with ease rather than anxiety.

Enhanced Creativity: When we open ourselves to change, we stimulate our creative faculties. Flexibility encourages us to view challenges as opportunities for growth and innovation. It breaks us free from the confines of conventional thinking and enables us to explore new possibilities. This creative liberation is not just beneficial for problem-solving in the workplace; it also translates into personal pursuits and passions.

Flexibility is a catalyst for creativity. When we embrace change, we open ourselves to a world of new possibilities and perspectives.

It's a dynamic process that stimulates creative thinking, allowing us to grow and innovate both personally and professionally.

New Perspectives: Flexibility encourages us to look at challenges and situations from different angles. This can lead to unique solutions and ideas that might not have been discovered through a rigid mindset.

Growth Mindset: A flexible approach fosters a growth mindset, where we see opportunities for development in every situation. This mindset is essential for personal and professional advancement.

Innovation: In the workplace, flexibility can lead to innovation. When teams are open to adapting their strategies and processes, they can create more effective and cutting-edge products and services.

By cultivating a flexible mindset, we can enhance our creative capacities, leading to a more balanced and enriched life.

Adaptability is not just about bending to the winds of change; it's about emerging stronger and more capable.

Individuals who embrace flexibility are better equipped to handle life's challenges and setbacks. They maintain motivation and perseverance, even in the face of adversity.

Improved Resilience: The ability to adapt is a hallmark of resilience. Adaptable individuals are not deterred by challenges or setbacks; instead, they find ways to maintain motivation and perseverance. This resilience is crucial in both professional and personal contexts, as it empowers us to recover from difficulties and continue pursuing our goals with renewed vigor.

Bouncing Back: Resilient individuals can recover from difficulties more quickly. They view setbacks as temporary and as opportunities for learning and growth.

Maintaining Motivation: When plans go awry, adaptable people can adjust their strategies and continue moving forward. Their motivation is not tied to a rigid path but to the achievement of their goals, however that may be accomplished.

Perseverance: Perseverance is the steadfastness in doing something despite difficulty or delay in achieving success. Flexible individuals persevere because they can find alternative routes to their destination.

Flexibility and resilience go hand in hand. By cultivating a flexible approach to life, we not only adapt to the present but also build the resilience needed to thrive in the future.

Recognize the Benefits of Flexibility in Work and Fitness Routines

Flexibility is the key to maintaining balance in our hectic lives. It allows us to adapt to the ebb and flow of daily demands without compromising our well-being. In work, it can mean the difference between a rigid schedule that leads to burnout and a dynamic one that fosters sustained productivity. In fitness, it enables us to keep moving forward, even when life throws obstacles in our path.

Flexibility is a crucial component in both work and fitness routines. It allows us to adapt to the ever-changing demands of our professional and personal lives, leading to improved productivity and health. By being flexible, we can better manage stress, increase our creativity, and build resilience against life's challenges.

Flexibility, therefore, is not just a strategy but a philosophy of life. It's about embracing the fluidity of our existence and finding the balance that allows us to thrive.

Implement Practical Strategies for Adapting to Changing Circumstances

Adaptability is not innate; it's a skill that can be developed with practice. By implementing strategies such as effective time management, exploring alternative workspaces, and adapting fitness routines, we can navigate life's uncertainties with confidence. These strategies empower us to remain productive and healthy, regardless of the circumstances.

Adapting to changing circumstances requires practical strategies that can be integrated into our daily lives. Techniques such as effective time management, exploring alternative workspaces, adapting fitness routines, and fostering a resilient mindset are essential for maintaining balance amidst life's uncertainties.

Cultivate a Mindset of Fluidity and Adaptability to Achieve Balance and Well-being

Ultimately, the goal is to cultivate a mindset that embraces change. This mindset is characterized by resilience, creativity, and an openness to new experiences. It's about seeing the potential in every situation and using it to our advantage.

With this approach, we can achieve a harmonious balance between our professional ambitions and personal health, leading to a richer, more fulfilling life.

A mindset of fluidity and adaptability is the foundation for achieving balance and well-being. It involves being open to new experiences, learning from change, and being willing to adjust our plans to maintain our commitment to our goals. This mindset not only helps us navigate the present but also prepares us for future success.

CHAPTER 4: MINDFUL TIME MANAGEMENT

- Incorporating mindfulness into time management practices.

- Balancing structured work time with mindful
breaks for physical activity.

- Strategies for prioritizing tasks and optimizing productivity.

Mindful Time Management

Effective time management is essential for maintaining productivity and achieving work-life balance. By incorporating mindfulness into our approach to time management, we can cultivate greater awareness and harmony in our daily routines.

Mindfulness is the practice of being fully present and engaged in the moment, aware of our thoughts and actions without judgment. When applied to time management, it transforms our relationship with time, making us more intentional about how we allocate our most precious resource.

Mindful Planning

Begin each day with a mindful planning session. Sit quietly and set intentions for the day. Reflect on your priorities and visualize accomplishing your tasks with calm and focus. This practice sets a purposeful tone for the day ahead.

Mindful Breaks

Take regular breaks to reset and recharge. Use these moments to step away from your work and engage in brief mindfulness exercises, such as deep breathing or a short walk. These breaks can boost your energy and enhance your focus.

Mindful Reflection

At the end of the day, spend a few minutes reflecting on your accomplishments and challenges. Acknowledge your efforts and learn from your experiences. This reflection helps you improve your time management skills over time.

1. Incorporating Mindfulness into Time Management Practices

Mindfulness is the practice of maintaining a nonjudgmental state of heightened or complete awareness of one's thoughts, emotions, or experiences on a moment-to-moment basis. When applied to time management, mindfulness becomes a powerful tool that can transform our relationship with time, tasks, and overall productivity.

Enhancing Focus: Mindfulness trains the brain to focus on the present task. This concentration can lead to deeper engagement with work, allowing for more efficient and high-quality output. Techniques like mindful breathing or focused attention on a single task can help anchor the mind, reducing the tendency to multitask and become distracted.

Mindfulness helps to train the brain to concentrate on the present moment. This heightened focus can lead to more efficient work, as you are fully engaged with the task at hand, minimizing distractions and maximizing productivity.

Techniques such as deep breathing exercises or mindful meditation can activate the body's relaxation response, counteracting the stress response.

Reducing Stress: The practice of mindfulness has been shown to lower stress levels. By bringing attention to the present and observing our thoughts without attachment, we can prevent the mind from spiraling into worries about the past or future.

Mindfulness techniques have been shown to reduce stress by helping individuals to remain calm and composed, especially in high-pressure situations. By focusing on the present, you can avoid becoming overwhelmed by future deadlines or past mistakes.

Promoting Better Decision-Making: Mindfulness enhances emotional regulation and cognitive flexibility, which are crucial for making informed decisions. With a clear mind, we can assess situations more objectively and choose actions that align with our goals and values. Body scans can be particularly useful in this regard, as they encourage a full awareness of our physical and emotional state, informing our decisions.

When you are mindful, you are able to observe your thoughts and emotions without getting caught up in them. This clear-headedness can lead to better decision-making, as you are able to consider all options objectively and choose the best course of action.

Techniques to Enhance Productivity and Well-being:

Deep Breathing: This technique involves taking slow, deep breaths to calm the mind and body. It can be done at the start of a work session or during breaks to refocus and reduce anxiety.

Body Scans: Starting from the toes and moving upwards, pay attention to each part of the body, noticing any sensations or tensions. This practice can lead to a greater awareness of stressors and the release of tension.

Present-Moment Awareness: Engage fully with the task at hand, noticing the details of the activity without judgment. This can be practiced during any routine task, such as eating lunch or walking to a meeting.

2. Balancing Structured Work Time with Mindful Breaks

Balancing structured work periods with mindful breaks is crucial for maintaining both productivity and well-being. Physical activity during these breaks plays a vital role in rejuvenating the body and mind, leading to sustained focus and creativity.

Pomodoro Technique: This technique involves working in short, focused intervals—traditionally 25 minutes—followed by a 5-minute break. These intervals, known as "pomodoros," are followed by longer breaks after every four cycles. The Pomodoro Technique helps maintain high levels of concentration while preventing fatigue. During the brief breaks, engaging in physical activity can help reset your mental state and keep the body energized.

Desk Stretches: Incorporating simple stretching exercises or yoga poses during breaks can significantly relieve tension and improve circulation, especially for those who spend long hours at a desk. Desk stretches can be done in a small space and without any equipment, making them an accessible option for most work environments.

Outdoor Walks: Taking mindful walks outdoors, even if just for a few minutes, can have a profound impact on mental clarity and creativity. The change of scenery, fresh air, and movement can help clear the mind and provide a new perspective on work-related challenges.

Deep Breathing: This involves taking slow, deliberate breaths to calm the mind and body, allowing for clearer thinking and better concentration.

Body Scans: This technique encourages awareness of different parts of the body, helping to identify and release any areas of tension or discomfort, which can improve focus and productivity.

Present-Moment Awareness: This practice involves focusing fully on the task at hand, observing every action and thought as it occurs, which can enhance performance and satisfaction with one's work.

By incorporating these mindfulness techniques into your time management practices, you can enhance your productivity and well-being, leading to a more balanced and fulfilling professional and personal life.

3. Strategies for Prioritizing Tasks and Optimizing Productivity

In the quest for productivity, it's not just about doing more—it's about doing what matters most. Here are some actionable strategies to prioritize tasks and optimize productivity:

Eisenhower Matrix: This time management tool helps categorize tasks based on their urgency and importance. It divides tasks into four quadrants:

Urgent and Important: Tasks that require immediate attention and have significant consequences.

Important but Not Urgent: Tasks that contribute to long-term goals and values but do not require immediate action.

Urgent but Not Important: Tasks that demand attention but do not contribute significantly to long-term goals.

Neither Urgent nor Important: Activities that offer little value and can often be eliminated.

By focusing on high-priority items first, particularly those in the "Important but Not Urgent" category, we can ensure that our efforts align with our most significant goals.

Time Blocking: This technique involves allocating specific time slots for different activities throughout the day. By scheduling time for work, exercise, rest, and personal pursuits, we create a structured yet flexible framework that can accommodate our priorities. Time blocking helps prevent overcommitment and ensures that each aspect of our lives receives the attention it deserves.

Single-Tasking: In contrast to multitasking, which can lead to decreased quality and increased stress, single-tasking promotes deep work and mindfulness. By focusing on one task at a time, we can improve our concentration and efficiency, leading to better outcomes and a greater sense of accomplishment.

Integrate Mindfulness Techniques into Daily Time Management Practices

Mindfulness techniques are essential for enhancing focus and reducing stress in our time management. By being fully present and engaged, we can manage our time more effectively and enjoy a more harmonious daily routine.

Incorporate Mindful Breaks for Physical Activity to Boost Energy and Focus

Mindful breaks, especially those involving physical activity, are vital for re-energizing the body and refocusing the mind. These breaks can lead to improved productivity and a better sense of well-being throughout the workday.

Implement Prioritization Strategies to Optimize Productivity and Well-being

Prioritization strategies, such as the Eisenhower Matrix and time blocking, help us focus on what's truly important. By optimizing our productivity through these methods, we can achieve our goals while maintaining our well-being.

Implementing these strategies can transform the way we approach our daily tasks, leading to a more mindful and productive life.

CHAPTER 5: INTEGRATING MOVEMENT INTO YOUR WORKDAY

- Creative ways to incorporate movement into sedentary work environments.

- Desk exercises, stretching routines, and mindful movement practices.

- Harnessing the power of micro-workouts for improved energy and focus.

In the modern workplace, where sedentary habits are the norm, integrating movement into your workday is vital for sustaining both physical health and mental well-being. This chapter will provide you with creative strategies and practical exercises to ensure you stay active, alert, and energized throughout your workday.

The Sedentary Challenge

The shift towards desk-bound jobs has led to a significant decrease in daily physical activity. The consequences of a sedentary lifestyle are far-reaching, affecting not just our physical health but also our mental acuity and emotional state.

Creative Strategies for Movement

Deskercise: Simple exercises that can be performed at your desk, such as seated leg lifts or desk push-ups, can keep the blood flowing without requiring a significant break from work.

Walking Meetings: Transform some of your meetings into walking ones. Not only does this incorporate movement, but the change of scenery can also spark creativity and engagement.

Active Commuting: Consider walking or cycling to work if possible. If you commute by public transport, get off a stop early and walk the rest of the way.

Standing Desks

Standing desks or adjustable workstations offer a simple yet effective solution to reduce sitting time. By alternating between sitting and standing, you can engage different muscle groups, improve posture, and increase circulation. The benefits include:

Reduced Risk of Chronic Diseases: Studies suggest that less sitting time can lower the risk of cardiovascular disease and diabetes.

Increased Energy: Standing can help reduce fatigue and increase energy levels, leading to more productive work sessions.

Engaged Muscles: Using a standing desk engages core and leg muscles, which can contribute to overall muscle tone and strength.

Active Meetings

Active meetings, such as walking meetings or stretching breaks during discussions, can make a significant difference. They not only promote physical activity but also encourage a more relaxed and open atmosphere for conversation. Benefits include:

Enhanced Creativity: Movement can stimulate creative thinking, potentially leading to more innovative ideas during discussions.

Improved Focus: Short physical breaks can help clear the mind, leading to improved focus and engagement in meetings.

Better Collaboration: Active meetings can break down formal barriers, fostering better collaboration and team dynamics.

Practical Exercises to Stay Active

Stretching Routine: Implement a series of stretches targeting the neck, back, and legs to combat the stiffness associated with prolonged sitting.

Mini-Circuits: Create a mini-circuit of bodyweight exercises, such as squats and lunges, to perform during longer breaks.

Stair Climbing: Opt for the stairs instead of the elevator. Regular stair climbing can improve cardiovascular health and increase leg strength.

Incorporating Movement Naturally

Stand More: Use a standing desk or set reminders to stand and move every hour.

Use Your Environment: Take advantage of any space available to you, whether it's a small office or a nearby park, to add some steps to your day.

Make It Fun: Incorporate elements of gamification, like setting daily step goals or having friendly competitions with colleagues.

Office Fitness Challenges

Office fitness challenges are a fun way to encourage colleagues to stay active. Whether it's a step competition, desk exercise routines, or a group fitness class, these challenges can promote a culture of health and camaraderie in the workplace. They offer:

Team Building: Challenges can strengthen team bonds and encourage a sense of community.

Motivation: Friendly competition can be a powerful motivator for individuals to increase their daily activity levels.

Health Awareness: Fitness challenges can raise awareness about the importance of physical activity and its impact on health and well-being.

Key Takeaways

Movement Matters: Regular movement throughout the day is crucial for physical and mental health.

Be Innovative: There are numerous ways to integrate movement into a sedentary workday; find what works best for your environment.

Make It Collective: Encouraging colleagues to participate in active initiatives can lead to a healthier, more engaged workplace.

By integrating these strategies into the workday, employees can combat the negative effects of a sedentary lifestyle, leading to improved health, increased energy, and greater overall well-being.

CHAPTER 6: DESIGNING ACTIVE WORK ENVIRONMENTS

- Strategies for creating workspaces that promote physical activity.

- Utilizing ergonomic tools, standing desks, and active seating options.

- Encouraging movement and collaboration within the workplace culture.

The design of our workspaces is a critical factor that influences our daily behaviors, health, productivity, and overall well-being. An active work environment is one that encourages movement, comfort, and collaboration, countering the sedentary nature of many modern workplaces.

In the contemporary world, productivity is not just about output—it's about our well-being. The design of our workspaces is a silent yet powerful contributor to our daily performance.

Strategies for Creating Active Workspaces

Ergonomic Furniture: Invest in adjustable desks and chairs that promote good posture and comfort. Ergonomic furniture can be tailored to the needs of each individual, reducing the risk of musculoskeletal disorders.

Dynamic Layouts: Design office layouts that encourage movement. This can include placing printers and other shared resources away from desks to encourage walking, or creating open spaces that invite spontaneous collaboration.

Natural Elements: Incorporate biophilic design principles by bringing elements of nature into the workspace. Plants, natural light, and outdoor views can reduce stress and enhance well-being.

Comfort in the workspace is not a luxury; it's a necessity. From temperature control to acoustic management, we'll examine how sensory experiences shape our ability to focus and produce high-quality work. Lighting plays a crucial role too—dynamic lighting systems that mimic natural light patterns can boost mood and energy levels.

The layout of a workspace can significantly influence the dynamics of teamwork. Open spaces, communal areas, and even the strategic placement of coffee machines can foster spontaneous interactions and idea exchanges. We'll look at design philosophies that encourage collaboration without sacrificing personal space.

Tools to Support Movement and Comfort

Sit-Stand Desks: Provide sit-stand desks that allow employees to easily switch between sitting and standing throughout the day. This can help reduce the negative health impacts of prolonged sitting.

Active Seating Options: Offer seating options like stability balls or active stools that engage core muscles and promote dynamic sitting.

Fitness Equipment: Consider having on-site fitness equipment such as treadmills or stationary bikes. Even small hand weights or resistance bands can be used for short exercise breaks.

In this digital age, the tools we use are integral to our workspaces. We'll review the latest in productivity software, from project management tools to apps that minimize distractions. Additionally, we'll consider the role of personal devices and how they can be integrated seamlessly into the active workspace.

To bring these concepts to life, we'll examine case studies of companies that have revolutionized their workspaces. We'll see firsthand the impact of these changes on employee satisfaction, health, and, ultimately, the bottom line.

Utilizing Ergonomic Tools, Standing Desks, and Active Seating Options

Ergonomic furniture and tools are designed to support the body's natural posture and reduce the risk of strain or injury. In this section, we delve into how these innovations can transform our workspaces and enhance productivity.

Standing Desks: Adjustable standing desks offer a dynamic workspace solution. By allowing users to easily switch between sitting and standing, these desks cater to the body's need for movement and can reduce the negative impacts of prolonged sitting, such as lower back pain and a sluggish metabolism.

Active Seating: Ergonomic chairs and balance balls are not just seating options; they're tools for wellness. These active seating solutions encourage micro-movements and core engagement, which can lead to improved posture, increased energy levels, and even heightened concentration.

Monitor Placement: The position of your monitor and keyboard is pivotal in creating an ergonomic workstation. Proper monitor height aligns with the user's natural line of sight, reducing neck strain, while an appropriately placed keyboard can minimize wrist pressure, preventing conditions like carpal tunnel syndrome.

By integrating these ergonomic tools into our daily routines, we can foster a workspace that promotes health, comfort, and, ultimately, a more sustainable form of productivity.

Encouraging Movement and Collaboration Within the Workplace Culture

Creating a vibrant and dynamic workplace culture is essential for fostering productivity and employee well-being. This section outlines strategies to promote a culture of movement and collaboration among team members.

Fitness Challenges: Workplace fitness challenges can be a fun and engaging way to build team spirit and encourage a healthy lifestyle. Organizing events like step-count competitions, cycling groups, or sports days can motivate employees to stay active and support each other's fitness goals.

Wellness Programs: Implementing wellness initiatives demonstrates a company's commitment to its employees' overall health. Offering yoga classes, meditation sessions, or access to onsite fitness facilities can make a significant difference in reducing stress, enhancing mental clarity, and promoting a sense of community within the workplace.

By integrating these practices, companies can cultivate an environment that values health and collaboration, leading to a more productive and satisfied workforce.

Implementing Movement-Friendly Design Principles

Objective: Enhance employee health and productivity through intentional design.

Spatial Layout: Discuss the importance of open spaces that encourage movement and interaction.

Natural Elements: Incorporate biophilic design principles to connect the workplace with nature, promoting mental and physical rejuvenation.

Flexibility: Advocate for adaptable workspaces that can be easily reconfigured for various activities and collaboration.

Investing in Ergonomic Tools and Furniture

Objective: Support optimal posture and comfort to improve work efficiency.

Ergonomic Assessment: Outline the process of evaluating the ergonomic needs of employees.

Investment Strategy: Provide guidance on selecting ergonomic tools and furniture that offer the best return on investment in terms of employee health and productivity.

Maintenance and Training: Emphasize the importance of maintaining ergonomic equipment and training staff on proper use to maximize benefits.

Fostering a Culture of Movement, Collaboration, and Well-being

Objective: Create a workplace environment that promotes holistic employee well-being.

Policy Development: Suggest policies that encourage regular breaks, physical activity, and social interaction.

Leadership Role: Explore how leadership can model and promote a culture of health and movement.

Community Building: Share ideas for creating a sense of community through wellness programs and team-building activities.

By addressing these key areas, businesses can redefine productivity to encompass not just output, but also the health and happiness of their employees.

CHAPTER 7: NOURISHING YOUR BODY AND MIND

- The role of nutrition in supporting both work performance and fitness goals.

- Mindful eating practices and strategies for maintaining energy levels throughout the day.

- Building a balanced plate for optimal nourishment and vitality.

The Foundation of Mindful Eating

In the hustle of meeting work deadlines and squeezing in gym sessions, nutrition often takes a backseat. Yet, it's the fuel that powers both our professional productivity and physical fitness. This chapter lays the groundwork for mindful eating—a practice that harmonizes our relationship with food and nourishes us wholly.

Building a Balanced Plate

A balanced plate is a canvas of nutrients that work in synergy to provide sustained energy and vitality. We'll dissect the components of a well-rounded meal:

Macronutrients: Understand the roles of carbohydrates, proteins, and fats in maintaining energy levels and supporting muscle recovery.

Micronutrients: Dive into the world of vitamins and minerals that bolster our immune system and enhance cognitive function.

Hydration: Learn about the importance of water in our diet and how it impacts every aspect of our well-being, from concentration to physical performance.

Mindful Eating in Practice

Transitioning from knowledge to action, we'll explore practical strategies for integrating mindful eating into a busy lifestyle:

Meal Planning: Tips for preparing balanced meals ahead of time to ensure you're nourished even on the busiest days.

Intuitive Eating: Encourage listening to your body's hunger and fullness cues to foster a healthy, guilt-free relationship with food.

Eating for Performance: Tailor your nutrition to support both your work and workout goals, ensuring that your body has the right fuel at the right time.

By the end of this chapter, readers will have a comprehensive understanding of how to nourish their bodies and minds, creating a sustainable foundation for success in all areas of life.

The Role of Nutrition in Supporting Work Performance and Fitness Goals

Nutrition is the cornerstone of both cognitive prowess and physical stamina. This section delves into how our dietary choices profoundly influence our work performance, fitness levels, and overall well-being.

Energy Levels: The foods we consume are directly linked to our energy reserves. Complex carbohydrates, lean proteins, and healthy fats provide a steady release of energy, fueling our bodies for the challenges of the day. We'll examine how to strategically choose foods that sustain energy levels from morning till night.

Recovery and Repair: Post-exercise nutrition is vital for muscle recovery and immune system support. Nutrients like protein and amino acids are the building blocks for repair, while antioxidants and vitamins help combat exercise-induced oxidative stress. This part of the chapter will highlight the key nutrients essential for a swift and effective recovery process.

Mental Clarity: A well-nourished brain is a foundation for sharp focus, enhanced memory, and a stable mood. Omega-3 fatty acids, B-vitamins, and iron play pivotal roles in cognitive health. We'll explore the brain-food connection and identify dietary patterns that support mental clarity and resilience against stress.

By understanding the integral role of nutrition in our professional and physical lives, we can make informed choices that elevate our performance across the board.

Mindful Eating Practices

Mindful eating is an approach that involves being fully present and engaged with the eating experience. It's about noticing the flavors, textures, and sensations of your food, as well as being aware of your body's hunger and fullness signals. This chapter will guide readers through the principles of mindful eating and how they can enhance overall well-being.

Eating with Awareness: We often eat on autopilot, not paying attention to what or how much we're consuming. This section encourages readers to tune into their body's cues for hunger and satiety. By doing so, one can avoid overeating and enjoy a more satisfying relationship with food.

Slow Eating: The act of chewing food thoroughly and taking the time to savor each bite is not only beneficial for digestion but also for appreciation of the meal. We'll discuss the importance of slowing down at mealtimes, which can lead to better digestion and increased satisfaction with smaller portions.

Emotional Eating Awareness: Emotions can have a significant impact on our eating habits. This part of the chapter addresses the common habit of emotional eating and provides strategies for recognizing and managing the emotions that trigger it. By cultivating awareness of emotional eating, readers can develop healthier responses to their emotions.

Through mindful eating practices, we can nourish our bodies and minds, leading to improved health, greater enjoyment of our meals, and a more balanced approach to nutrition.

Strategies for Maintaining Energy Levels Throughout the Day

Maintaining steady energy levels is crucial for both productivity and fitness. This section provides practical tips for constructing balanced meals and choosing smart snacks that support sustained energy throughout the day.

Balanced Plate: A balanced meal is like a symphony, where each nutrient plays a crucial role in sustaining energy. Here's how to create harmony on your plate:

Proteins: Build and repair tissues with lean meats, legumes, and dairy.

Carbohydrates: Fuel your day with whole grains, fruits, and vegetables.

Fats: Support cell growth and hormone production with nuts, seeds, and avocados.

Fiber: Regulate digestion and keep full longer with leafy greens and whole grains.

Smart Snacking: Smart snacking is about choosing foods

that satisfy hunger while providing nutritional value:

Nuts and Seeds: A handful of almonds or sunflower seeds can provide a quick protein and healthy fat boost.

Greek Yogurt: Rich in protein and probiotics, it's a smart choice for a midday snack.

Fresh Fruit: An apple or banana offers natural sugars for a quick energy lift and fiber for sustained release.

Hydration: Water is the elixir of life and a key player in maintaining energy levels:

Start Your Day with Water: Begin with a glass of water to kickstart your metabolism.

Consistent Intake: Keep a water bottle at your desk and take regular sips throughout the day.

Hydration Before Caffeine: Choose water over caffeinated beverages when you first feel tired.

By incorporating these strategies into your daily routine, you can ensure that your body and mind are well-nourished, leading to enhanced performance in all areas of life.

Understanding Nutrition's Impact

Objective: Comprehend the influence of nutrition on work, fitness, and well-being.

Cognitive Function: Explore how nutrition affects focus, decision-making, and productivity.

Physical Performance: Examine the role of diet in fitness achievements and recovery.

Holistic Health: Consider how a balanced diet contributes to overall health and longevity.

Practicing Mindful Eating

Objective: Enhance meal satisfaction and self-awareness.

Awareness Techniques: Learn to recognize hunger and fullness cues.

Mindful Habits: Slow down and savor the flavors and textures of food.

Emotional Intelligence: Understand the connection between emotions and eating patterns.

Building Balanced Meals and Snacks

Objective: Maintain energy and promote health throughout the day.

Meal Composition: Create meals with a mix of macronutrients for sustained energy.

Snacking Wisely: Choose snacks that provide energy and nutrients without the crash.

Staying Hydrated: Recognize the importance of water for cognitive and physical performance.

By integrating these principles, readers can foster a nourishing lifestyle that supports their professional ambitions and personal health goals.

CHAPTER 8: FINDING JOY IN MOVEMENT

- The role of nutrition in supporting both work performance and fitness goals.

- Mindful eating practices and strategies for maintaining energy levels throughout the day.

- Building a balanced plate for optimal nourishment and vitality.

Rediscovering the Joy of Physical Activity

Movement is an essential expression of life, a celebration of what our bodies can do. This chapter is an invitation to step away from the rigid routines and rediscover the intrinsic joy that comes from being active. It's about finding pleasure in movement and making it a cherished part of our daily lives.

Playful Pursuits: Engaging in activities that feel like play can transform our perspective on exercise. Whether it's dancing, hiking, playing a sport, or even a game of tag with your kids, playful pursuits make physical activity something to look forward to, not a chore to check off.

Personalized Activities: There is no one-size-fits-all when it comes to enjoying movement. This section encourages readers to explore a variety of activities to find what truly resonates with them. It's about personal preference, whether that means yoga, martial arts, swimming, or cycling.

The Fulfillment Factor: Beyond the physical benefits, engaging in enjoyable activities provides a sense of accomplishment and fulfillment. We'll explore how setting personal goals and celebrating achievements, no matter how small, can enhance the joy of movement.

By the end of this chapter, readers will have a renewed appreciation for the role of physical activity in their lives, not just for health, but for happiness and fulfillment.
Rediscovering the Joy of Movement

Physical activity is more than a means to an end; it's a journey to joy and self-discovery. This section celebrates the intrinsic rewards of movement that extend far beyond fitness metrics.

Playful Activities: Life is meant to be enjoyed, and so is movement. We encourage readers to find joy in activities that make them smile. Whether it's the rhythm of dancing, the adventure of hiking, the freedom of cycling, or the camaraderie of team sports, playful activities can uplift the spirit and invigorate the body.

Mind-Body Connection: Movement is a powerful form of self-expression and a pathway to inner peace. It's a dialogue between the body and the soul. This chapter highlights how activities like martial arts, dance, or even a simple stretch can serve as tools for stress relief, fostering a state of emotional well-being.

Connection with Nature: Immersing ourselves in the natural world is a reminder of our place in the larger tapestry of life. Outdoor activities like walking in lush parks, practicing yoga under the open sky, or simply taking a moment to breathe in the fresh air can deepen our connection with nature, enhancing our sense of well-being and grounding us in the present moment.

By embracing these practices, we nourish not just our bodies, but our minds and spirits, finding joy in every step, stretch, and stride.

Exploring Various Forms of Exercise and Movement

Embracing a variety of exercises can enrich our fitness journey and cater to our unique preferences and goals. This section encourages readers to explore the diverse world of physical activity.

Fitness Diversity: The realm of fitness is vast and varied, offering something for everyone. From the tranquility of yoga to the intensity of strength training, the discipline of martial arts to the exuberance of dance, each modality brings its own benefits and joys. We'll introduce a spectrum of exercise options to inspire readers to find their fit.

Personalized Approach: The key to a sustainable fitness routine is personal enjoyment and suitability. This chapter advocates for experimentation with different activities to discover what resonates most with you. It's about listening to your body and choosing activities that align with your interests, fitness level, and lifestyle.

Social Engagement: Group fitness classes and team sports offer more than just physical benefits; they provide a sense of community and shared purpose. We'll highlight how social engagement in exercise can boost motivation, accountability, and enjoyment, making the path to fitness a collective and rewarding experience.

By exploring and embracing the variety of exercises available, readers can craft a personalized and enjoyable fitness routine that supports both their body and mind.

Cultivating a Mindset of Curiosity and Exploration in Fitness

Pursuits

Adopting a mindset of curiosity and exploration can transform the fitness journey into an enriching experience of personal growth and discovery. This section provides insights on fostering such a mindset.

Growth Mindset: Physical activity is more than a routine; it's an opportunity for self-discovery and improvement. We encourage readers to embrace challenges and view each workout as a chance to learn something new about their abilities and potential. It's not about perfection, but progress and the willingness to step out of comfort zones.

Overcoming Barriers: Many face mental hurdles like self-doubt or fear of judgment that can impede their fitness journey.

This chapter addresses these common barriers and offers strategies to overcome them:

Self-Reflection: Identify the root of these fears and confront them with positive affirmations.

Small Steps: Start with manageable goals to build confidence and momentum.

Supportive Community: Seek out groups or partners who provide encouragement and share similar goals.

Celebrating Progress: Recognizing and celebrating each milestone, no matter how small, is crucial for motivation and self-appreciation. Whether it's lifting a heavier weight, running an extra mile, or simply sticking to a routine, every achievement is a step forward in the journey of fitness and should be celebrated.

By cultivating a mindset of curiosity and exploration, individuals can find deeper meaning in their fitness pursuits, leading to a more fulfilling and sustained practice.

Prioritizing Enjoyment and Fulfillment

Emphasize the importance of joy in physical activity over strict fitness regimens.

Personal Fulfillment: Encourage readers to find activities that bring them happiness and satisfaction.

Flexible Goals: Advocate for adaptable fitness objectives that accommodate life's ebb and flow.

Experimenting with Diverse Forms of Exercise

Discover personal resonance through varied fitness experiences.

Exploration of Activities: Introduce a wide range of exercises to suit different preferences and abilities.

Personalized Fitness: Guide readers to tailor their exercise choices to their unique lifestyle and interests.

Cultivating a Mindset of Curiosity and Growth

Objective: Foster a perspective of self-discovery and continuous improvement in fitness.

Growth-Oriented Approach: Inspire a mindset that views challenges as opportunities for growth.

Overcoming Mental Barriers: Provide strategies to navigate common psychological obstacles in fitness.

Celebrating Every Step: Highlight the significance of acknowledging and celebrating progress, no matter the size.

CHAPTER 9: CULTIVATING RESTORATIVE PRACTICES

- The importance of rest and recovery in achieving work-fitness balance.

- Incorporating restorative practices such as yoga, meditation, and breathwork into your routine.

- Prioritizing sleep hygiene for optimal physical and mental well-being.

The Art of Rest and Recovery

In our fast-paced world, rest is often undervalued, yet it's a critical element of a holistic health approach. This chapter delves into the restorative practices that replenish our energy reserves and promote healing on all levels.

Physical Rejuvenation: We'll explore techniques such as:

Sleep Hygiene: Strategies for improving sleep quality and quantity, recognizing sleep as the foundation of physical recovery.

Active Recovery: Gentle movement practices like yoga or tai chi that facilitate physical restoration while keeping the body engaged.

Mental and Emotional Rejuvenation: Techniques to soothe the mind and uplift the spirit, including:

Mindfulness Meditation: Practices to enhance present-moment awareness and reduce stress.

Digital Detox: Encouraging regular intervals away from screens and technology to reset the mind.

Integrating Restorative Practices: Practical tips for incorporating these techniques into daily life, such as:

Routine Setting: Establishing a restorative routine that aligns with individual lifestyles and needs.

Environment Design: Creating a personal space conducive to relaxation and rejuvenation.

By the end of this chapter, readers will have a comprehensive understanding of the importance of rest and recovery and be equipped with the tools to implement restorative practices into their lives, leading to improved health and well-being.

The Art of Rest and Recovery

In our fast-paced world, rest is often undervalued, yet it's a critical element of a holistic health approach. This chapter delves into the restorative practices that replenish our energy reserves and promote healing on all levels.

Physical Rejuvenation: We'll explore techniques such as:

Sleep Hygiene: Strategies for improving sleep quality and quantity, recognizing sleep as the foundation of physical recovery.

Active Recovery: Gentle movement practices like yoga or tai chi that facilitate physical restoration while keeping the body engaged.

Mental and Emotional Rejuvenation: Techniques to soothe the mind and uplift the spirit, including:

Mindfulness Meditation: Practices to enhance present-moment awareness and reduce stress.

Digital Detox: Encouraging regular intervals away from screens and technology to reset the mind.

Integrating Restorative Practices: Practical tips for incorporating these techniques into daily life, such as:

Routine Setting: Establishing a restorative routine that aligns with individual lifestyles and needs.

Environment Design: Creating a personal space conducive to relaxation and rejuvenation.

Incorporating Restorative Practices into Your Routine

In the quest for health and vitality, restorative practices are as vital as any workout. They are the yin to the yang of our active lives, providing the necessary balance through relaxation and renewal.

Yoga and Stretching: Gentle yoga poses and stretching routines are the perfect antidote to the tension that accumulates in our bodies. We'll explore:

Poses: Such as Child's Pose and Cat-Cow, which are known for their tension-releasing properties.

Routines: A series of stretches that can be done in just a few minutes to improve flexibility and circulation.

Meditation and Mindfulness: The mind, like the body, needs time to rest and recover. Techniques to calm the mind include:

Guided Meditation: Using audio guides to lead you through relaxation and visualization exercises.

Mindfulness Exercises: Simple practices that can be integrated into daily life, such as mindful walking or eating.

Breathwork: The breath is a powerful tool for regulating the body's stress response. We'll teach:

Techniques: Like deep diaphragmatic breathing, which can be used anytime to promote relaxation and reduce stress.

Practices: Incorporating breathwork into your daily routine to maintain a state of calm and balance.

By making these restorative practices a regular part of your routine, you can support your body's natural healing processes and cultivate a deep sense of well-being.

Prioritizing Sleep Hygiene

Good sleep hygiene is essential for our physical, mental, and emotional health. This section offers guidance on optimizing both the quality and quantity of sleep for overall well-being.

Creating a Conducive Sleep Environment: A restful night's sleep starts with the right environment. Consider these elements:

Comfortable Mattress and Pillows: Ensure your bed is supportive and comfortable.

Darkness: Use blackout curtains or an eye mask to block out light.

Quiet: Reduce noise with earplugs or a white noise machine.

Temperature: Keep the room cool, ideally between 60-67 degrees

Fahrenheit.

Establishing Calming Bedtime Rituals: Bedtime rituals signal to your body that it's time to wind down. Here are some activities to try:

Reading: Engage in a light read that doesn't overstimulate the brain.

Soothing Music: Listen to calm tunes or nature sounds to relax your mind.

Breathing Exercises: Practice deep breathing or progressive muscle relaxation to ease into sleep.

Maintaining a Consistent Sleep Schedule: Regularity is key for a healthy sleep cycle.

Fixed Wake-Up Time: Wake up at the same time every day, even on weekends.

Pre-Sleep Routine: Start your bedtime routine at the same time each night.

Circadian Rhythms: Align your sleep schedule with natural light patterns when possible.

> By prioritizing sleep hygiene, you can enhance your sleep quality, which in turn, can improve your daily functioning and overall quality of life.

CHAPTER 10: FOSTERING SUPPORTIVE COMMUNITIES

- Building a network of like-minded individuals who prioritize both work and fitness.

- Finding accountability partners and support systems to stay motivated and inspired.

- Creating a culture of wellness within your personal and professional circles.

The Power of Connection

Human beings are social creatures, and the communities we build play a pivotal role in our motivation, accountability, and overall well-being. This chapter explores the art of creating and nurturing supportive communities that share a commitment to both professional success and personal health.

Building Connections: We'll discuss strategies for connecting with like-minded individuals:

Networking Events: Attend industry conferences, workshops, and fitness expos to meet peers.

Social Media Groups: Join online forums and groups focused on work-life balance and fitness.

Local Clubs: Become a member of local sports clubs or co-working spaces that value health and productivity.

Nurturing Relationships: Once connections are made, it's important to foster them:

Regular Meetups: Organize or participate in regular meetups to maintain engagement.

Shared Goals: Collaborate on common objectives, such as group fitness challenges or professional projects.

Support Systems: Create a system of support where members can turn to each other for advice, encouragement, and accountability.

Community Benefits:

Highlight the benefits of being part of a supportive community:

Motivation: Draw inspiration from the achievements and dedication of community members.

Accountability: Stay on track with your goals through mutual accountability.

Well-Being: Enhance your overall well-being by being part of a group that understands and supports your dual priorities of work and fitness.

By the end of this chapter, readers will have a blueprint for cultivating communities that enrich their professional and personal lives, creating a synergy that fuels success in both arenas.

Building a Network of Like-Minded Individuals

The journey towards balancing work and fitness is enriched when shared with others who understand and support your goals. This section highlights the benefits of cultivating a network of like-minded individuals.

Shared Motivation: Surrounding yourself with individuals who share your values and aspirations can be incredibly motivating. A supportive community acts as a catalyst for commitment, pushing you to stay true to your work and fitness goals. It's the collective energy and shared vision that keep you inspired and driven.

Knowledge Sharing: A network of peers is a treasure trove of collective wisdom. Exchanging ideas, experiences, and resources can lead to new insights and strategies for managing work and fitness. Whether it's a productivity hack or a workout tip, the knowledge shared within a community is invaluable.

Social Connection: Beyond the practical benefits, the social connection itself is vital for mental and emotional well-being. It provides a sense of belonging and support that can buffer against stress and isolation. Engaging with a community can enrich your life with meaningful relationships and a sense of camaraderie.

By building and nurturing a network of like-minded individuals, you can enjoy a more fulfilling journey towards achieving a harmonious balance between your professional ambitions and personal health objectives.

Finding Accountability Partners and Support Systems

The path to balancing work and fitness is often smoother with a reliable support system. This section outlines the importance of finding accountability partners and engaging with supportive networks.

Accountability Buddies: Partnering with an accountability buddy can be a game-changer. It's about having someone to share your goals with, who will:

- Encourage you on tough days.

- Provide feedback on your progress.

- Help maintain accountability for mutual goals.

Online Communities: The digital age offers a plethora of virtual platforms where like-minded individuals gather. These online communities can be a rich resource for:

- Sharing experiences and tips.

- Gaining motivation from others' successes.

- Finding support during challenging times.

Professional Networks: Engaging with colleagues or industry peers who also prioritize health can lead to:

- Collaborative wellness initiatives within the workplace.

- Networking opportunities that align professional growth with personal health.

- Mentorship in navigating the intersection of career advancement and fitness.

By actively seeking out and participating in these supportive environments, individuals can enhance their journey towards a balanced lifestyle, enriched by the camaraderie and shared wisdom of their peers.

Creating a Culture of Wellness Within Your Circles

Promoting a culture of wellness in our personal and professional lives not only benefits us individually but also strengthens the communities we are part of. This section explores actionable ways to foster this culture.

Organize Wellness Activities: Taking the initiative to organize group activities can significantly enhance engagement and camaraderie. Consider these ideas:

Group Workouts: Whether it's a running club or a group yoga session, shared physical activities can be both fun and motivating.

Wellness Challenges: Set up challenges like hydration weeks or step-count competitions to encourage healthy habits.

Healthy Cooking Sessions: Share recipes and cook together, either virtually or in person, to promote nutritious eating.

Lead by Example: Your actions can inspire others to prioritize their health and well-being. Here's how you can lead by example:

Work-Fitness Balance: Show how you integrate fitness into your busy schedule.

Wellness Advocacy: Share your experiences and the benefits you've observed from living a balanced lifestyle.

Cultivate Positive Relationships: Relationships that are supportive and uplifting can have a profound impact on our growth and well-being. To cultivate such relationships:

Encourage Open Dialogue: Create an environment where discussions about health and wellness are welcomed.

Offer Support: Be there for others in their wellness journey, offering encouragement and celebrating their successes.

By implementing these strategies, you can contribute to

creating a supportive atmosphere that values and promotes wellness, leading to healthier, happier individuals and stronger communities.

Recognizing the Power of Community

Objective: Understand the role of community in enhancing work-fitness balance and overall wellness.

Community Influence: Explore how a supportive community can positively impact our motivation and well-being.

Shared Experiences: Discuss the benefits of shared experiences and goals within a community setting.

Seeking Accountability Partners and Support Systems

Objective: Find individuals or groups that provide motivation and inspiration.

Accountability Mechanisms: Outline the importance of accountability in maintaining commitment to goals.

Support Networks: Identify different types of support systems, from personal connections to professional networks.

Contributing to a Culture of Wellness

Objective: Actively participate in promoting wellness in various circles.

Initiating Wellness Activities: Suggest ways to engage others in wellness practices.

Leading by Example: Encourage personal commitment to wellness as a means to inspire others.

Positive Relationship Building: Emphasize the importance of

fostering relationships that support mutual growth and well-being.

By embracing these concepts, readers can leverage the strength of community to foster a supportive environment that encourages a balanced approach to work and fitness.

CHAPTER 11: EMBRACING SELF-COMPASSION

- Practicing self-compassion in the face of setbacks and challenges.

- Letting go of perfectionism and embracing imperfection as part of the journey.

- Celebrating progress and small victories along the way.

Embracing Self-Compassion

Cultivating Resilience and Inner Peace

In the pursuit of balancing work and fitness, it's crucial to practice self-compassion. This chapter explores the transformative power of self-compassion as a tool for resilience, motivation, and inner peace.

Understanding Self-Compassion: At its core, self-compassion is about treating oneself with the same kindness and understanding that we would offer to a good friend. It involves three key components:

- Self-Kindness: Replace self-criticism with a more nurturing and understanding voice.

- Common Humanity: Recognize that imperfection and setbacks are part of the shared human experience.
- Mindfulness: Be present with your experiences without judgment or denial.

Practices to Foster Self-Compassion:

We'll introduce practical ways to cultivate self-compassion:

- Self-Compassion Breaks: Take moments throughout the day to offer yourself kindness and understanding.
- Gratitude Journaling: Reflect on and write down things you're grateful for, including aspects of yourself and your achievements.

- Affirmations: Use positive affirmations to reinforce self-compassion and counter negative self-talk.

Mindset Shifts for Self-Compassion: Adopting a self-compassionate mindset can lead to profound changes in how we approach our goals and challenges:

Growth Mindset: Embrace challenges as opportunities for growth rather than signs of failure.

Forgiveness: Learn to forgive yourself for setbacks and view them as learning experiences.

Patience: Give yourself the time you need to grow and achieve your goals without harsh timelines.

By embracing self-compassion, we can navigate the journey

toward work-fitness balance with greater ease and kindness towards ourselves, leading to a more fulfilling and peaceful life.

Practicing Self-Compassion in the Face of Setbacks and Challenges

When we encounter setbacks and challenges, it's essential to navigate these moments with self-compassion. This section underscores the importance of treating ourselves with kindness and understanding during difficult times.

Self-Kindness: It's easy to be our own harshest critic, but self-kindness is a more constructive response. We encourage readers to:

Offer Empathy: Extend the same compassion to yourself that you would to a friend.

Positive Self-Talk: Replace critical thoughts with supportive and affirming messages.

Forgiveness: Allow yourself to make mistakes and learn from them without harsh judgment.

Common Humanity: Setbacks are a universal aspect of the human experience. Emphasizing this can help readers:

Feel Connected: Understand that they are not alone in facing difficulties.

Normalize Challenges: Accept that obstacles are a natural part of life's journey.

Share Experiences: Open up about struggles to foster connection and support.

Mindful Awareness: Cultivating a non-judgmental awareness of our thoughts and emotions is key to self-compassion. We'll explore practices to:

- Observe Without Judgment: Recognize thoughts and feelings without labeling them as good or bad.

- Stay Present: Engage with the current moment without dwelling on past errors or future worries.

- Self-Reflection: Use mindfulness to gain insights into personal patterns and behaviors.

Letting Go of Perfectionism and Embracing Imperfection

Perfectionism can be a double-edged sword. While it drives us to achieve high standards, it can also lead to self-defeating thoughts and behaviors. This section discusses the drawbacks of perfectionism and the liberating benefits of embracing imperfection.

Growth Mindset: Instead of viewing setbacks as failures, we encourage readers to adopt a growth mindset:

Learning Opportunities: See mistakes as valuable lessons that contribute to personal development.

Progress Over Perfection: Focus on continuous improvement rather than an unattainable ideal.

Flexibility and Adaptability: Life is unpredictable, and rigid adherence to perfection can be limiting. We emphasize:

- Adjusting Goals: Be willing to modify your objectives as situations change.

- Resilience: Develop the ability to bounce back from challenges with a flexible approach.

Embracing Vulnerability: Authenticity and vulnerability are strengths, not weaknesses. We advocate:

- Self-Acceptance: Recognize and accept your imperfections as part of your unique journey.

- Sharing Experiences: Connect with others by sharing your challenges and how you've overcome them.

By letting go of perfectionism and embracing imperfection, we open ourselves to a more authentic, fulfilling, and compassionate way of living and working.

Celebrating Progress and Small Victories Along the Way

Acknowledging and celebrating every step forward is essential for maintaining motivation and a positive outlook. This section provides strategies for recognizing and honoring personal achievements, no matter their size.

Milestone Reflection: Regular reflection on progress helps to build a sense of accomplishment and purpose. We encourage readers to:

- Keep a Progress Journal: Document milestones, no matter how small, and reflect on the journey.

- Share Achievements: Discussing progress with friends, family, or community members can amplify the sense of achievement.

Gratitude Practice: Cultivating gratitude for the journey enriches the experience of growth and evolution. Consider:

Daily Gratitude: Start or end your day by listing things you're grateful for, including your own efforts and progress.

- Gratitude Reminders: Set reminders to pause and appreciate the moment and your hard work throughout the day.

Self-Celebration Rituals: Creating personal rituals to celebrate achievements can reinforce positive behaviors and boost self-esteem. Some ideas include:

Reward System: Set up a system to reward yourself for reaching milestones, whether it's a treat, a break, or a special activity.

Victory Dance: Have a go-to celebration dance or gesture for when you accomplish a goal.

Celebration Circle: Gather with friends or community members to celebrate each other's victories.

By embracing these practices, readers can create a rewarding cycle of setting goals, achieving them, and celebrating, which fuels further progress and personal growth.

CHAPTER 12: SUSTAINING BALANCE FOR THE LONG RUN

- Strategies for maintaining work-fitness balance over the long term.

- Embracing a mindset of sustainability and moderation in work and fitness pursuits.

- Setting boundaries and priorities to preserve overall well-being.

Maintaining Equilibrium in Work and Fitness

Achieving a balance between work and fitness is not a one-time task but a continuous process that evolves with our changing lives. This chapter provides insights into maintaining this balance over the long term, emphasizing well-being and moderation.

Intentional Strategies for Balance: We'll explore various strategies to maintain balance:

- Time Management: Effective scheduling techniques to allocate time for both work and fitness without compromising either.

- Priority Setting: Learning to prioritize tasks and activities that align with your long-term health and career goals.

- Flexibility: Being adaptable to life's changes and willing to adjust your balance strategies as needed.

Mindful Practices for Well-Being: Mindfulness is key to sustaining balance:

- Mindful Exercise: Engaging in physical activity with full awareness to enhance its benefits and enjoyment.

- Work Mindfulness: Applying mindfulness at work to improve focus and reduce stress.

- Self-Care Routines: Incorporating regular self-care practices that support both mental and physical health.

Moderation as a Philosophy:

Living in moderation helps prevent burnout and ensures sustainability:

- Balanced Workload: Avoiding overcommitment at work and setting realistic expectations.

- Moderate Fitness Goals: Setting achievable fitness goals that promote health without leading to exhaustion.

- Rest and Recovery: Ensuring adequate rest and recovery time to prevent overtraining and work-related stress.

By embracing these principles, readers can create a sustainable approach to balancing their professional and personal lives, leading to lasting well-being and satisfaction.

Strategies for Maintaining Work-Fitness Balance Over the Long Term

Maintaining a work-fitness balance is an ongoing process that requires dedication and strategic planning. This section outlines practical approaches to sustain this balance over time.

Consistent Routine: Establishing a regular schedule is foundational to maintaining balance. Consider these elements:

- Work Schedule: Set clear boundaries for work hours to prevent overworking.

- Exercise Time: Block out consistent times for physical activity, making it as routine as brushing your teeth.

- Rest Periods: Schedule downtime to relax and recharge, just as you would any other important appointment.

- Personal Time: Ensure you have moments in the day dedicated to hobbies, family, and self-care.

Flexibility and Adaptability:

While consistency is key, so is the ability to adapt. Life is full of unexpected changes, and our routines should be able to accommodate them:

- Adjust as Needed: Be prepared to modify your routine in response to life's demands.

- Resilient Mindset: Cultivate resilience by viewing challenges as opportunities to grow and learn.

- Stay Focused: Keep your overall balance in mind, even when making adjustments.

Goal Setting: Setting goals gives you direction and motivation. To ensure they are sustainable, remember to:

- Be Realistic: Set goals that are achievable and won't lead to burnout.

- Align with Values: Make sure your goals reflect your long-term health and well-being priorities.

- Review Regularly: Revisit and adjust your goals as your circumstances and priorities evolve.

By implementing these strategies, you can create a balanced lifestyle that supports both your career ambitions and personal health over the long haul.

Embracing a Mindset of Sustainability and Moderation

A balanced and sustainable approach to work and fitness is key to long-term success and well-being. This section encourages readers to adopt practices that promote sustainability and moderation.

Avoiding Burnout: Burnout can derail even the most dedicated individuals. To prevent it, we must:

- Recognize the Signs: Be aware of burnout symptoms such as chronic fatigue, irritability, and reduced performance.

- Prioritize Self-Care: Implement self-care routines that recharge your mind and body, like hobbies, relaxation techniques, and social activities.

- Set Boundaries: Establish clear boundaries between work and personal time to ensure you have space to unwind.

Allowing for Rest: Rest is not a luxury; it's a necessity for resilience. It's important to:

Value Recovery Time: Understand that rest is crucial for physical repair and mental clarity.

- Incorporate Rest Days: Schedule regular days off from both work and exercise to fully recover.

- Listen to Your Body: Pay attention to what your body is telling you and rest when needed, not just when scheduled.

Enjoying the Journey: Shifting the focus from outcomes to the process can lead to a more fulfilling experience:

- Process Over Outcome: Find joy in the daily activities and small improvements, not just the end goals.

- Celebrate Learning: Embrace new learnings and experiences as part of the growth process.

- Stay Present: Focus on the present moment and the task at hand, rather than constantly looking ahead to the next achievement.

By embracing these principles, you can enjoy a more balanced journey toward your work and fitness goals, one that is sustainable and moderated for long-term health and happiness.

Setting Boundaries and Priorities to Preserve Overall Well-being

In the pursuit of success and fulfillment, it's easy to lose sight of the delicate balance that sustains our well-being. This chapter is dedicated to empowering you, the reader, to establish boundaries and prioritize your overall health and happiness.

Saying No: The Power of a Positive Refusal

Learning to say no is an essential skill in maintaining balance. It's about recognizing that saying yes to everything often means saying no to your own well-being. This section will explore strategies to:

- Identify when a request is in conflict with your well-being.

- Communicate your refusal assertively yet respectfully.

- Understand that saying no can lead to better opportunities that align with your personal and professional goals.

Protecting Personal Time: Your Sanctuary of Rejuvenation

Personal time is non-negotiable. It's the period during which you recharge and find peace away from the demands of the world. In this part, we'll delve into:

- Creating a personal time schedule that's sacred and non-intrusive.

- Activities that can significantly enhance your relaxation and rejuvenation.

- The importance of hobbies and social connections in creating a well-rounded life.

Aligning Values: Steering Life with Your Inner Compass

Your core values are the guiding stars of your life's journey. Aligning your actions with these values ensures a path of integrity and satisfaction. This segment will provide insights on:

- Reflecting on what truly matters to you and how to make decisions that reflect these priorities.

- Setting goals that resonate with your deepest convictions.

- Living a life that feels authentic and fulfilling by honoring your personal values.

Conclusion: Harmonizing Work and Fitness for a Fulfilling Life

- Reflecting on the journey of integrating work
and fitness into a harmonious lifestyle.

- Encouragement to continue prioritizing both
aspects for sustained well-being.

- Final thoughts and actionable steps for
achieving holistic balance in life.

As we culminate our exploration of balancing work and fitness, it's time to embrace the lessons learned and the strides made towards a more integrated and fulfilling life. This chapter serves as a reflection and a guide to solidify the practices that foster a harmonious existence.

The Transformative Journey

The path to harmonizing work and fitness is not a destination but a continuous journey. It's about making conscious choices every day that contribute to your overall well-being. This section will encourage readers to:

Reflect on the progress made and the habits formed.

Recognize the importance of consistency and the small steps that lead to significant changes.

Celebrate the victories, no matter how small, and learn from the setbacks without self-judgment.

Mindfulness: The Anchor of Balance

Mindfulness is the practice of being present and fully engaged with whatever we're doing at the moment — free from distraction or judgment, and aware of our thoughts and feelings without getting caught up in them. This chapter will delve into:

Techniques to cultivate mindfulness in daily activities, especially during work and exercise.

The benefits of mindfulness in reducing stress and enhancing performance.

How to apply mindfulness to maintain a balance between professional ambitions and personal health.

Self-Compassion: The Heart of the Matter

At the core of a balanced life is self-compassion. It's about treating yourself with the same kindness and understanding that you would offer to a good friend. In this final section, we'll explore:

The role of self-compassion in overcoming obstacles and maintaining motivation.

Strategies for practicing self-compassion when facing challenges in work and fitness goals.

The impact of self-compassion on mental health and its ripple effect on every aspect of life.

By integrating the principles of dedication, mindfulness, and self-compassion, this chapter aims to fortify the reader's commitment to a life where work and fitness coexist in harmony, leading to a more satisfying and holistic well-being.

Reflecting on the Journey

As we draw the curtains on this chapter of our lives, it's a moment to pause and look back at the path we've treaded in aligning work and fitness. This reflection is not just about acknowledging the distance covered but also about appreciating the transformation within.

Acknowledging Progress

Progress is not measured solely by the milestones reached but also by the habits cultivated along the way. This section will guide readers through:

Recognizing the small yet significant lifestyle changes that have contributed to better health.

Understanding the importance of consistency and the cumulative effect of daily self-care practices.

Embracing the journey of self-improvement as an ongoing process rather than a finite goal.

Celebrating Challenges and Lessons

Every challenge faced is an opportunity for growth. Celebration is a form of gratitude for the strength and wisdom gained. In this part, we'll discuss:

How to find joy in the challenges overcome and the resilience built.

The lessons learned from each obstacle and how they pave the way for future success.

The art of transforming setbacks into comebacks and leveraging experiences for personal development.

Recognizing the Impact

The balance between work and fitness has a profound impact on our overall well-being. This segment will focus on:

The tangible benefits of a balanced lifestyle on physical health and mental clarity.

The positive ripple effects on happiness, relationships, and professional productivity.

Strategies to maintain and improve this balance, ensuring a lasting and fulfilling life.

Through introspection and celebration, this chapter aims to solidify the reader's commitment to a life where work and fitness are not at odds but in harmony, enhancing the quality of life and leading to enduring satisfaction and success.

Encouragement for Sustained Prioritization

In the symphony of life, the harmonious blend of work and fitness plays a crucial melody. As we continue to compose our lives, the following verses serve as an encouragement to sustain the prioritization of both these essential elements.

Embrace the Journey

Life is a journey—a tapestry woven with threads of various experiences, challenges, and triumphs. To embrace this journey means to:

Accept that self-improvement is a lifelong endeavor, not limited by time or age.

Recognize that holistic balance is the key to a vibrant and fulfilling life.

Commit to continuous learning and growth, understanding that each day offers a new opportunity to enhance our well-being.

Stay Motivated

Motivation is the wind beneath the wings of our aspirations. To stay aloft, we must:

Reflect on the myriad benefits that a balanced lifestyle brings to our health, happiness, and productivity.

Celebrate every milestone, no matter how small, and let it fuel our journey forward.

Visualize the future we wish to create and let that vision drive our daily actions.

Build Your Community

Community is the chorus that supports the soloist on stage. To amplify our efforts, we should:

Surround ourselves with people who share our commitment to a balanced life.

Engage with accountability partners who help us stay on track and remind us of our goals.

Participate in groups that inspire and challenge us to reach new heights in both our professional and personal lives.

This chapter is a call to action—a reminder that the balance between work and fitness is not just a goal to be achieved but a lifestyle to be lived. It's an invitation to continue prioritizing these aspects for a life of sustained well-being and growth.

Final Thoughts and Actionable Steps

As we conclude this guide to a balanced life, let's anchor ourselves with actionable steps that will serve as the foundation for a journey filled with purpose, health, and joy.

Setting Realistic Goals

Realistic goals are the beacons that guide us through the fog of daily demands. They provide clarity and direction. This section will help readers:

Define clear, achievable objectives that align with personal capabilities and resources.

Break down larger goals into smaller, manageable tasks to prevent overwhelm.

Establish routines that integrate work and fitness seamlessly into daily life.

Practicing Self-Compassion

Self-compassion is the gentle reminder that we are human and perfection is not the goal. This part of the chapter will focus on:

Techniques to practice kindness towards oneself during moments of struggle.

The importance of recognizing and accepting imperfections as natural steps in the process of growth.

Strategies to reframe setbacks as learning opportunities rather than failures.

Cultivating Gratitude

Gratitude is the soil in which joy and contentment grow. It transforms our perspective and enhances our life experience. In this segment, we'll explore:

Daily practices to cultivate a sense of gratitude for the present moment.

The impact of gratitude on mental well-being and its ability to amplify positive emotions.

Ways to express gratitude towards oneself and others, fostering a supportive and uplifting environment.

By embracing these final thoughts and actionable steps, you are setting the stage for a life where work and fitness are not competing forces but synergistic elements that enrich your existence. Carry these lessons forward and let them guide you to a life of balance, growth, and fulfillment.

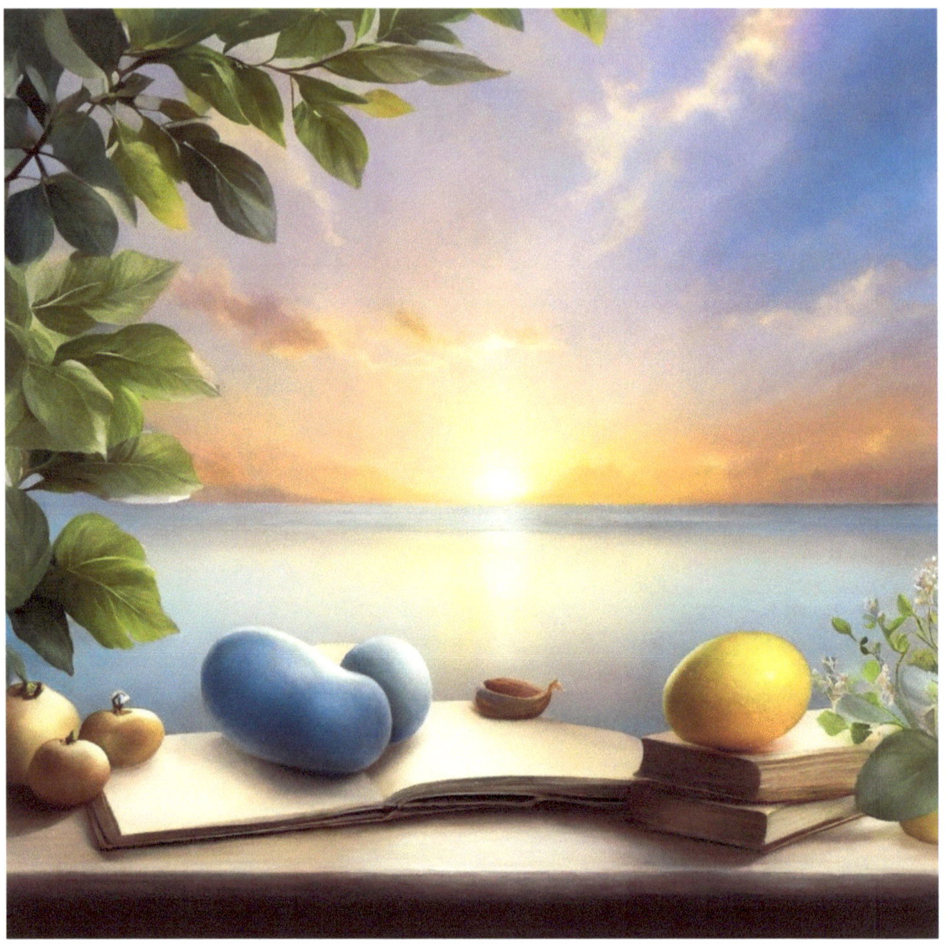